DOCTOR BARBARA SIMPLE 7-DAY JUICE DETOX

Revitalize your health with Dr. Barbara's 7-days juice detox, discover simple, effective recipes for cleaning, rejuvenation and optimal health

I0774146

Charlos Luz

Table of Contents

COPYRIGHT © 2023

All rights reserved. No part of this publication may be reproduced, distributed, or transmitted in any form or by any means, including photocopying, recording, or other electronic or mechanical methods, without the prior written permission of the publisher, except in the case of brief quotations embodied in critical reviews and certain other noncommercial uses permitted by copyright law.

CHAPTER ONE

Introduction to Doctor Barbara's Detox Method: Understanding the Principles of Herbal Juicing for Cleansing

In a world where health trends come and go, there's one method that has stood the test of time: detoxification. The concept of detoxifying the body to rid it of harmful toxins and improve overall health has been around for centuries. Among the myriad of detox methods available, herbal juicing stands out as a natural and effective way to cleanse the body. In this comprehensive guide, we delve into the principles behind Doctor Barbara's Detox Method, focusing on the use of herbal juices for cleansing purposes.

Understanding Detoxification: The Body's Natural Process

Before diving into the specifics of herbal juicing, it's essential to understand the process of detoxification and its significance for overall health. Detoxification is the body's natural mechanism for eliminating toxins and waste products that accumulate from various sources such as environmental pollutants, processed foods, and metabolic byproducts.

The body has several organs involved in the detoxification process, including the liver, kidneys, lungs, skin, and lymphatic system. These organs work together to neutralize and eliminate toxins through processes like metabolism, filtration, and excretion. However, in today's modern world filled with pollutants and unhealthy lifestyle choices, the body's natural detoxification pathways can become overwhelmed, leading to a buildup of toxins and potential health issues.

The Role of Herbal Juicing in Detoxification

Herbal juicing has gained popularity as a holistic approach to detoxification, offering a natural and effective way to support the body's cleansing processes. Unlike commercial detox programs that may rely on restrictive diets or harsh cleansing protocols, herbal juicing harnesses the power of plant-based nutrients to nourish and detoxify the body gently.

The principle behind herbal juicing for detoxification lies in the abundance of vitamins, minerals, antioxidants, and phytonutrients found in fresh fruits, vegetables, and herbs. These nutrients play vital roles in supporting the body's detox pathways, enhancing liver function, promoting cellular repair, and boosting immune function.

Doctor Barbara's Detox Method: A Holistic Approach

Doctor Barbara's Detox Method is a holistic approach to cleansing and rejuvenating the body using a combination of herbal juices, dietary modifications, and lifestyle practices. Founded on the principles of natural healing and wellness, this method aims to restore balance and vitality to the body by supporting its inherent detoxification processes.

Central to Doctor Barbara's Detox Method is the use of freshly prepared herbal juices made from organic fruits, vegetables, and herbs. These juices are carefully selected for their detoxifying properties and blended to create synergistic combinations that enhance their effectiveness. By consuming these nutrient-dense juices, participants provide their bodies with an abundance of vitamins, minerals, enzymes, and antioxidants needed for optimal detoxification and rejuvenation.

Key Principles of Herbal Juicing in Doctor Barbara's Detox Method

1. **Organic Ingredients**: Doctor Barbara's Detox Method emphasizes the use of organic produce to minimize exposure to pesticides, herbicides, and other harmful chemicals that can negate the detoxification process.

2. **Variety and Balance**: The method encourages a diverse selection of fruits, vegetables, and herbs to ensure a broad spectrum of nutrients and phytochemicals that support detoxification pathways.

3. **Hydration and Cleansing**: Herbal juices act as natural diuretics, helping to flush out toxins from the body while

providing essential hydration to support cellular function and metabolic processes.

4. **Alkalizing and Energizing**: Many of the ingredients used in herbal juices have alkalizing properties, helping to balance the body's pH levels and promote energy production, which is crucial for optimal detoxification.

5. **Supporting Liver Function**: The liver plays a central role in detoxification, and certain herbs such as dandelion, milk thistle, and turmeric are known for their ability to support liver health and enhance detoxification pathways.

6. **Gentle Elimination**: Unlike harsh cleanses that may cause discomfort or disruption to normal bodily functions, Doctor Barbara's Detox Method focuses on gentle and gradual detoxification, allowing the body to cleanse naturally without undue stress.

Implementation and Guidelines for Herbal Juicing

Implementing Doctor Barbara's Detox Method involves a structured approach to herbal juicing, dietary modifications, and lifestyle practices. Participants are typically guided through a specific protocol that may include:

1. **Preparation Phase**: Before starting the detox program, participants may be advised to gradually reduce the intake of

processed foods, caffeine, alcohol, and other dietary toxins to prepare the body for cleansing.

2. **Juice Recipes**: Doctor Barbara's Detox Method provides a variety of juice recipes tailored to support different aspects of detoxification, such as liver support, kidney cleansing, or immune boosting. These recipes often include a combination of fruits, vegetables, and herbs known for their detoxifying properties.

3. **Juicing Schedule**: Participants are instructed to consume multiple servings of herbal juices throughout the day, ideally on an empty stomach to maximize absorption and detoxification benefits.

4. **Hydration and Herbal Teas**: In addition to herbal juices, participants are encouraged to stay hydrated by drinking plenty of water and herbal teas that support detoxification and enhance elimination.

5. **Supplementation**: Depending on individual needs, supplements such as probiotics, digestive enzymes, or specific herbal extracts may be recommended to support detoxification and overall health.

6. **Incorporating Whole Foods**: While herbal juicing is a central component of the detox program, participants are also encouraged to incorporate whole foods such as salads,

steamed vegetables, and lean proteins to ensure adequate nutrition and support ongoing detoxification.

Benefits of Doctor Barbara's Detox Method

1. **Improved Digestion**: Herbal juicing and dietary modifications can help improve digestion by providing essential nutrients, enzymes, and fiber that support gastrointestinal health and regularity.

2. **Increased Energy and Vitality**: Detoxification removes the burden of toxins from the body, allowing for improved energy production, mental clarity, and overall vitality.

3. **Weight Management**: By promoting the elimination of waste and supporting metabolic function, Doctor Barbara's Detox Method may help individuals achieve and maintain a healthy weight.

4. **Enhanced Immune Function**: The abundance of vitamins, minerals, and antioxidants in herbal juices strengthens the immune system, helping the body defend against infections and illness.

5. **Radiant Skin and Hair**: Detoxification supports cellular repair and regeneration, leading to clearer skin, shinier hair, and an overall youthful appearance.

6. **Mental and Emotional Clarity**: Many participants report experiencing increased mental clarity, focus, and emotional

balance as a result of detoxification, which can positively impact overall well-being.

Conclusion

In conclusion, Doctor Barbara's Detox Method offers a holistic and effective approach to cleansing the body using herbal juicing as a central component. By understanding the principles behind detoxification and the role of herbal juices in supporting this process, individuals can embark on a journey towards improved health, vitality, and well-being. Whether seeking to boost energy levels, support digestion, or enhance overall wellness, Doctor Barbara's Detox Method provides a comprehensive framework for achieving optimal health through natural and sustainable means.

CHAPTER TWO

The Importance of Detoxification: Exploring How Toxins Accumulate in the Body and Impact Health

In today's modern world, our bodies are constantly bombarded with toxins from various sources, including pollution, processed foods, household chemicals, and stress. These toxins can accumulate in our bodies over time, potentially leading to a wide range of health issues. Understanding the importance of detoxification is crucial for maintaining optimal health and well-being. In this comprehensive exploration, we'll delve into how toxins accumulate in the body, their impact on health, and the significance of detoxification in mitigating these effects.

Toxins: The Silent Threat

Toxins are substances that can harm the body's cells, tissues, and organs, disrupting normal physiological functions and contributing to disease. They come in various forms, including heavy metals, environmental pollutants, pesticides, food additives, and metabolic waste products. While the body has natural detoxification mechanisms to eliminate these toxins, the sheer volume and complexity of toxins in our environment can overwhelm these processes, leading to toxin buildup and adverse health effects.

Sources of Toxins

Toxins can enter the body through multiple routes, including:

1. **Air**: Pollution from vehicle exhaust, industrial emissions, and indoor pollutants like cigarette smoke can introduce toxins into the respiratory system and bloodstream.

2. **Food and Water**: Pesticides, herbicides, preservatives, and contaminants like heavy metals can contaminate food and water sources, exposing the digestive system to toxins.

3. **Personal Care Products**: Skincare products, cosmetics, and hygiene products often contain chemicals like parabens, phthalates, and synthetic fragrances that can be absorbed through the skin and enter the bloodstream.

4. **Household Cleaners**: Cleaning products, air fresheners, and other household chemicals release toxins into the air, which can be inhaled or absorbed through the skin.

5. **Plastics**: Plastics contain harmful chemicals like bisphenol-A (BPA) and phthalates, which can leach into food, water, and the environment, posing a risk of toxin exposure.

6. **Stress**: Chronic stress can trigger the release of stress hormones like cortisol, which, when elevated over time, can have toxic effects on the body and contribute to inflammation and disease.

The Impact of Toxins on Health

Toxins can wreak havoc on virtually every system of the body, leading to a myriad of health problems, including:

1. **Immune Dysfunction**: Toxins can suppress immune function, making the body more susceptible to infections, allergies, and autoimmune disorders.

2. **Inflammation**: Many toxins trigger inflammation in the body, contributing to chronic diseases such as arthritis, cardiovascular disease, and cancer.

3. **Hormonal Imbalance**: Endocrine-disrupting chemicals (EDCs) found in certain toxins can interfere with hormone production and regulation, leading to reproductive issues, thyroid disorders, and metabolic imbalances.

4. **Neurological Disorders**: Some toxins, such as heavy metals and pesticides, can cross the blood-brain barrier and impair neurological function, increasing the risk of cognitive decline, neurodevelopmental disorders, and mood disorders.

5. **Organ Damage**: Toxins can accumulate in organs such as the liver, kidneys, and lungs, impairing their function and contributing to organ damage, dysfunction, and disease.

6. **Cancer Risk**: Certain toxins are carcinogenic and can damage DNA, disrupt cellular function, and promote the development of cancerous tumors.

The Body's Natural Detoxification Mechanisms

Fortunately, the body has built-in mechanisms for detoxification to help neutralize and eliminate toxins, including:

1. **Liver Detoxification**: The liver is the body's primary detoxification organ, responsible for metabolizing toxins and converting them into water-soluble compounds that can be excreted via urine or bile.

2. **Kidney Filtration**: The kidneys filter waste products and toxins from the blood, excreting them in the form of urine.

3. **Lymphatic System**: The lymphatic system helps remove toxins and waste products from tissues and transports them to lymph nodes for elimination.

4. **Digestive System**: The digestive tract plays a role in detoxification by breaking down food and absorbing nutrients while eliminating waste products and toxins through bowel movements.

5. **Skin Detoxification**: Sweat glands in the skin help eliminate toxins through perspiration, making regular exercise and saunas beneficial for detoxification.

The Importance of Supporting Detoxification

While the body has innate detoxification mechanisms, they can become overwhelmed or compromised due to toxin overload, poor diet, sedentary lifestyle, and other factors. Therefore, supporting detoxification through healthy lifestyle practices is essential for maintaining optimal health and well-being. Key strategies for supporting detoxification include:

1. **Nutrient-Rich Diet**: Consuming a diet rich in fruits, vegetables, whole grains, and lean proteins provides essential nutrients and antioxidants that support detoxification pathways.

2. **Hydration**: Drinking plenty of water helps flush toxins from the body and supports kidney function.

3. **Regular Exercise**: Physical activity promotes circulation, lymphatic drainage, and sweating, facilitating the elimination of toxins from the body.

4. **Stress Management**: Practicing stress-reduction techniques such as meditation, deep breathing, and yoga helps lower cortisol levels and support detoxification.

5. **Limiting Toxin Exposure**: Minimizing exposure to environmental toxins by choosing organic foods, using natural personal care products, and reducing exposure to pollution and household chemicals.

6. **Detoxification Protocols**: Periodic detox programs, such as herbal cleanses or juice fasts, can support the body's natural detoxification processes and promote toxin elimination.

Conclusion

In conclusion, the importance of detoxification cannot be overstated in today's toxin-laden world. Toxins accumulate in the body from various sources and can have detrimental effects on health, ranging from immune dysfunction and inflammation to organ damage and cancer. Supporting the body's natural detoxification mechanisms through healthy lifestyle practices is essential for mitigating the effects of toxins and maintaining optimal health and well-being. By understanding how toxins accumulate in the body and the impact they have on health, individuals can take proactive steps to support detoxification and promote overall wellness.

CHAPTER THREE

Doctor Barbara's Philosophy on Herbal Juicing: Harnessing the Healing Power of Fresh, Nutrient-Dense Juices

Doctor Barbara's philosophy on herbal juicing revolves around the belief in the inherent healing power of fresh, nutrient-dense juices derived from organic fruits, vegetables, and herbs. Founded on principles of holistic health and natural healing, this philosophy emphasizes the vital role that herbal juices play in nourishing the body, supporting detoxification, and promoting overall wellness. In this comprehensive exploration, we delve into the key tenets of Doctor Barbara's philosophy on herbal juicing and how it harnesses the healing potential of nature's bounty.

The Healing Power of Plants

Central to Doctor Barbara's philosophy is the recognition of the healing properties found in plants. Throughout history, various cultures have utilized herbs and botanicals for their medicinal properties, harnessing the therapeutic benefits of phytonutrients, antioxidants, vitamins, and minerals found abundantly in nature. Herbal juicing allows for the concentrated extraction of these healing compounds, making them readily available for absorption and utilization by the body.

Nutrient Density and Bioavailability

Doctor Barbara emphasizes the importance of nutrient density and bioavailability in herbal juicing. Unlike processed foods and supplements, which may contain synthetic additives and lack the full spectrum of nutrients found in whole foods, fresh juices are rich in vitamins, minerals, enzymes, and phytonutrients in their natural, bioavailable forms. This nutrient density ensures that the body receives an abundance of essential nutrients necessary for optimal health and vitality.

Supporting Detoxification and Cleansing

Herbal juicing plays a crucial role in supporting the body's natural detoxification and cleansing processes. The liver, kidneys, lungs, skin, and lymphatic system work tirelessly to eliminate toxins and waste products from the body, but modern lifestyles and environmental exposures can overwhelm these detoxification pathways. By providing the body with a concentrated source of detoxifying nutrients, herbal juices aid in the elimination of toxins while nourishing and revitalizing cells and tissues.

Alkalizing and Balancing pH Levels

Many of the ingredients used in herbal juices have alkalizing properties, which help balance the body's pH levels and support overall health. An acidic internal environment can contribute to inflammation, oxidative stress, and disease, whereas alkaline-forming foods and beverages help neutralize acidity and promote a more alkaline state. Herbal juices rich in alkalizing fruits, vegetables, and herbs help maintain the body's acid-base balance, creating an environment conducive to healing and vitality.

Synergistic Blends for Optimal Health

Doctor Barbara emphasizes the importance of creating synergistic blends of fruits, vegetables, and herbs in herbal juices to maximize their therapeutic benefits. Each ingredient is carefully selected for its unique properties and combined to create harmonious blends that enhance detoxification, support organ function, boost immunity, and promote overall well-being. By leveraging the synergistic interactions between different plant compounds, herbal juices deliver comprehensive nourishment and healing to the body.

Embracing Organic and Sustainable Practices

In alignment with principles of natural health and environmental stewardship, Doctor Barbara advocates for the use of organic and sustainable ingredients in herbal juicing. Organic produce is free from synthetic pesticides, herbicides, and fertilizers, minimizing exposure to harmful chemicals and maximizing the nutritional quality of juices. Additionally, supporting sustainable farming practices helps preserve soil health, biodiversity, and ecological balance for future generations.

Holistic Approach to Wellness

Doctor Barbara's philosophy on herbal juicing extends beyond mere nutrition to encompass a holistic approach to wellness. Recognizing the interconnectedness of body, mind, and spirit, this philosophy emphasizes the importance of lifestyle factors such as stress management, adequate sleep, physical activity, and emotional well-being in supporting overall health. Herbal juicing serves as one component of a comprehensive wellness regimen, complementing other health-promoting practices to foster holistic balance and vitality.

Conclusion

In conclusion, Doctor Barbara's philosophy on herbal juicing embodies a deep reverence for the healing power of nature and a commitment to holistic health and wellness. By harnessing the nutrient-rich bounty of organic fruits, vegetables, and herbs, herbal juicing offers a potent means of nourishing the body, supporting detoxification, and promoting vitality. Through synergistic blends, alkalizing properties, and sustainable practices, herbal juicing serves as a cornerstone of a holistic approach to wellness, empowering individuals to cultivate optimal health and vitality from the inside out.

CHAPTER FOUR

Preparing for the Detox: Guidelines for Pre-Cleanse Preparation and Transitioning to Juicing

Embarking on a detox journey, particularly one centered around herbal juicing like Doctor Barbara's Detox Method, requires careful preparation and transition to ensure optimal results and minimize discomfort. Preparing the body and mind for the detox process is essential for maximizing its effectiveness and supporting overall well-being. In this guide, we provide comprehensive guidelines for pre-cleanse preparation and transitioning to juicing to help individuals embark on their detox journey with confidence and success.

Understanding Pre-Cleanse Preparation

Pre-cleanse preparation involves taking proactive steps to prepare the body and mind for the detox process ahead. This phase typically focuses on gradually reducing dietary toxins, hydrating the body, and mentally preparing for the cleanse. The goals of pre-cleanse preparation include:

1. **Reducing Toxin Load**: Gradually reducing consumption of processed foods, caffeine, alcohol, sugar, and other dietary toxins helps minimize the toxin load on the body and ease the transition into the cleanse.

2. **Hydration**: Drinking plenty of water and herbal teas helps hydrate the body, support kidney function, and flush out toxins, preparing the body for the increased fluid intake during the cleanse.

3. **Nutrient-Rich Diet**: Emphasizing whole, nutrient-rich foods such as fruits, vegetables, whole grains, and lean proteins provides essential nutrients and antioxidants that support detoxification pathways and overall health.

4. **Mental Preparation**: Mentally preparing for the cleanse involves setting intentions, visualizing success, and cultivating a positive mindset to support commitment and perseverance throughout the detox process.

Guidelines for Pre-Cleanse Preparation

1. **Gradual Transition**: Begin reducing intake of processed foods, caffeine, alcohol, and sugar at least 1-2 weeks before starting the cleanse. Gradually increase consumption of fruits, vegetables, whole grains, and lean proteins to support detoxification and nourish the body.

2. **Hydration**: Drink at least 8-10 glasses of water per day to stay hydrated and support kidney function. Incorporate herbal teas such as dandelion root, ginger, or green tea to aid in detoxification and hydration.

3. **Nutrient-Rich Foods**: Focus on consuming a diet rich in fruits, vegetables, whole grains, nuts, seeds, and legumes to provide essential nutrients and antioxidants that support detoxification and overall health.

4. **Eliminate Trigger Foods**: Identify and eliminate potential trigger foods such as dairy, gluten, soy, and processed foods that may contribute to inflammation, digestive issues, or food sensitivities.

5. **Supportive Supplements**: Consider incorporating supportive supplements such as probiotics, digestive enzymes, and herbal extracts (e.g., milk thistle, dandelion root) to support detoxification pathways and optimize overall health.

6. **Mindful Eating**: Practice mindful eating habits, such as chewing food thoroughly, eating slowly, and paying attention to hunger and fullness cues, to enhance digestion and nutrient absorption.

Transitioning to Juicing

Transitioning to juicing involves gradually introducing herbal juices into the diet while phasing out solid foods. This gradual transition helps acclimate the body to the cleanse, reduces potential detox symptoms, and supports optimal nutrient absorption. Here are guidelines for transitioning to juicing:

1. **Start Slow**: Begin by replacing one meal per day with a herbal juice, such as breakfast or lunch, while continuing to consume balanced meals for the remaining meals.

2. **Increase Frequency**: Gradually increase the frequency of juicing over several days, replacing additional meals with herbal juices until you are consuming primarily juices.

3. **Hydration**: Continue to drink plenty of water and herbal teas throughout the day to stay hydrated and support detoxification.

4. **Listen to Your Body**: Pay attention to how your body responds to the transition to juicing. If you experience digestive discomfort or detox symptoms, such as headaches or fatigue, consider slowing down the transition or adjusting the types of juices consumed.

5. **Variety**: Incorporate a variety of herbal juices made from different fruits, vegetables, and herbs to ensure a broad spectrum of nutrients and phytochemicals that support detoxification and overall health.

6. **Mind-Body Practices**: Engage in mind-body practices such as meditation, deep breathing, yoga, or gentle exercise to reduce stress, support relaxation, and enhance the detoxification process.

Conclusion

Preparing for a detox involves thoughtful planning, gradual transition, and mindful awareness of the body's needs. By following guidelines for pre-cleanse preparation and transitioning to juicing, individuals can set themselves up for a successful and rewarding detox experience. Through gradual reduction of dietary toxins, hydration, nutrient-rich foods, and mindful eating, the body is primed to embrace the healing power of herbal juicing and embark on a journey toward renewed health and vitality.

CHAPTER FIVE

The 7-Day Herbal Juice Detox Protocol: Step-by-Step Instructions for Daily Juicing and Hydration

Embarking on a 7-day herbal juice detox can be a transformative journey towards renewed health, vitality, and well-being. With careful planning and dedication, participants can support their body's natural detoxification processes, nourish cells with essential nutrients, and experience a renewed sense of energy and vitality. In this comprehensive guide, we provide step-by-step instructions for each day of the detox protocol, outlining daily juicing routines, hydration guidelines, and tips for optimizing the detox experience.

Day 1: Preparation and Mindset

1. **Morning**: Start the day with a glass of warm water with lemon to kickstart digestion and hydration. Set intentions for the detox journey, focusing on renewal, vitality, and self-care.

2. **Breakfast**: Enjoy a light and nourishing breakfast such as overnight oats topped with fresh berries or a green smoothie made with spinach, banana, and almond milk.

3. **Lunch**: Incorporate a colorful salad with mixed greens, vegetables, and a protein source such as grilled chicken or

chickpeas. Avoid heavy or processed foods to ease the transition into the detox.

4. **Afternoon**: Prepare for the detox by stocking up on organic fruits, vegetables, and herbs for juicing. Cleanse the kitchen and juicer to ensure a hygienic juicing environment.

5. **Dinner**: Keep dinner light with a vegetable-based soup or broth accompanied by a side of steamed vegetables. Avoid caffeine, alcohol, and processed foods to support detoxification.

6. **Evening**: Take time for relaxation and self-care activities such as gentle stretching, meditation, or a warm bath to promote restful sleep and prepare for the detox journey ahead.

Day 2-7: Daily Juicing and Hydration Protocol

Morning Routine:

1. **Hydration**: Upon waking, drink a large glass of water or herbal tea to hydrate the body and kickstart metabolism.

2. **Herbal Juice**: Prepare a fresh herbal juice using a combination of organic fruits, vegetables, and herbs chosen for their detoxifying properties. Examples include:

   - Green Detox Juice: Spinach, cucumber, celery, green apple, lemon, and ginger.

- Liver Cleanse Juice: Beetroot, carrot, apple, lemon, and dandelion greens.

- Immune Booster Juice: Orange, carrot, turmeric, ginger, and pineapple.

3. **Breakfast**: Enjoy a light and balanced breakfast to complement the herbal juice, such as overnight oats, chia pudding, or a fruit smoothie bowl topped with nuts and seeds.

Midday Routine:

1. **Hydration**: Continue to drink water, herbal teas, or coconut water throughout the morning to stay hydrated and support detoxification.

2. **Herbal Juice**: Consume another serving of herbal juice mid-morning or as a midday snack to maintain hydration and nourishment.

3. **Light Meal**: Opt for a light and nutrient-dense meal for lunch, such as a salad with leafy greens, vegetables, avocado, and a lean protein source. Avoid heavy or processed foods that may hinder detoxification.

Afternoon Routine:

1. **Hydration**: Drink herbal teas, infused water, or coconut water to stay hydrated and support detoxification throughout the afternoon.

2. **Herbal Juice**: Enjoy another serving of herbal juice in the afternoon to replenish nutrients and support energy levels.

3. **Snack**: Incorporate a light and healthy snack such as raw vegetables with hummus, fresh fruit, or a handful of nuts and seeds to satisfy hunger and provide sustained energy.

Evening Routine:

1. **Hydration**: Hydrate with water or herbal teas in the evening to support detoxification and promote relaxation.

2. **Dinner**: Keep dinner light and plant-based, focusing on steamed or lightly cooked vegetables, whole grains, and legumes. Avoid heavy or rich foods that may disrupt digestion or sleep.

3. **Evening Ritual**: Wind down with a calming evening ritual such as gentle yoga, meditation, or journaling to promote relaxation and prepare for restful sleep.

Additional Tips for Success:

1. **Stay Hydrated**: Drink plenty of water, herbal teas, and coconut water throughout the day to stay hydrated and support detoxification.

2. **Listen to Your Body**: Pay attention to hunger cues, energy levels, and any signs of discomfort or detox symptoms. Adjust your juicing and meal plan accordingly to meet your body's needs.

3. **Supportive Supplements**: Consider incorporating supportive supplements such as probiotics, digestive enzymes, or herbal extracts to enhance detoxification and support overall health.

4. **Rest and Relaxation**: Prioritize restful sleep, stress management, and self-care activities to support the body's natural healing processes and optimize the detox experience.

5. **Gradual Transition**: Ease back into solid foods gradually after completing the detox, starting with light, plant-based meals and gradually reintroducing other foods as tolerated.

By following this comprehensive 7-day herbal juice detox protocol, participants can support their body's natural detoxification processes, nourish cells with essential nutrients, and experience a renewed sense of vitality and well-being. With careful planning, dedication, and mindfulness, the detox journey can be a transformative experience towards optimal health and vitality.

CHAPTER SIX

Selecting the Right Herbs: Identifying Key Ingredients for Detoxifying Herbal Juices

Choosing the right herbs is crucial for creating detoxifying herbal juices that support the body's natural cleansing processes and promote overall well-being. Incorporating a variety of herbs with detoxifying properties can enhance the effectiveness of herbal juices and provide a diverse array of nutrients and phytochemicals. In this guide, we identify key ingredients for detoxifying herbal juices and explore their specific benefits for supporting detoxification and promoting optimal health.

1. Dandelion

Dandelion is a potent detoxifying herb known for its liver-cleansing properties. Rich in antioxidants and bitter compounds, dandelion stimulates bile production, aiding in the digestion and elimination of toxins from the liver and gallbladder. Incorporating dandelion leaves or roots into herbal juices can support liver function, promote detoxification, and enhance overall health.

2. Milk Thistle

Milk thistle is another powerful herb renowned for its liver-protective and detoxifying properties. The active compound in milk thistle, silymarin, helps regenerate liver cells, protect against liver damage, and support the liver's detoxification processes.

Including milk thistle extract or seeds in herbal juices can help support liver health, reduce inflammation, and enhance detoxification.

3. Turmeric

Turmeric is a vibrant yellow spice prized for its anti-inflammatory, antioxidant, and detoxifying properties. Curcumin, the active compound in turmeric, helps stimulate bile production, enhance liver function, and promote detoxification pathways. Adding fresh turmeric root or powdered turmeric to herbal juices can support liver health, reduce inflammation, and aid in detoxification.

4. Ginger

Ginger is a warming and invigorating herb with potent detoxifying and digestive benefits. Gingerol, the active compound in ginger, helps stimulate digestion, support liver function, and alleviate digestive discomfort. Incorporating fresh ginger root or ginger juice into herbal juices can aid in digestion, reduce nausea, and support detoxification.

5. Parsley

Parsley is a nutrient-rich herb that provides an array of vitamins, minerals, and antioxidants essential for detoxification and overall health. Rich in chlorophyll and flavonoids, parsley helps support kidney function, promote urinary tract health, and eliminate toxins from the body. Including fresh parsley leaves or parsley juice in herbal juices can support detoxification, reduce inflammation, and promote overall wellness.

6. Cilantro

Cilantro, also known as coriander, is a flavorful herb with potent detoxifying properties. Cilantro contains compounds that help bind to heavy metals and facilitate their elimination from the body. Incorporating fresh cilantro leaves or cilantro juice into herbal juices can support heavy metal detoxification, reduce oxidative stress, and promote overall health.

7. Lemon

Lemon is a cleansing and alkalizing citrus fruit rich in vitamin C and antioxidants. Lemon helps stimulate digestion, support liver function, and promote detoxification by enhancing bile production and aiding in the elimination of toxins from the body. Adding fresh lemon juice or lemon zest to herbal juices can enhance flavor, promote hydration, and support detoxification.

8. Beetroot

Beetroot is a vibrant root vegetable packed with nutrients and phytochemicals that support detoxification and overall health. Betalains, the pigments responsible for beetroot's deep red color, have been shown to support liver function, reduce inflammation, and enhance detoxification pathways. Incorporating fresh beetroot juice or beetroot powder into herbal juices can support liver health, improve blood circulation, and promote detoxification.

9. Wheatgrass

Wheatgrass is a nutrient-rich superfood known for its detoxifying and alkalizing properties. Packed with chlorophyll, vitamins, minerals, and antioxidants, wheatgrass helps support liver function, enhance detoxification, and promote overall vitality. Incorporating fresh wheatgrass juice or wheatgrass powder into herbal juices can support cellular detoxification, boost energy levels, and enhance overall health.

10. Spirulina

Spirulina is a nutrient-dense blue-green algae rich in protein, vitamins, minerals, and antioxidants. Spirulina helps support detoxification by binding to heavy metals and toxins in the body and aiding in their elimination. Incorporating spirulina powder into herbal juices can support immune function, reduce inflammation, and promote detoxification.

By incorporating these key herbs into herbal juices, individuals can create potent detoxifying blends that support the body's natural cleansing processes, promote optimal health, and enhance overall well-being. Experimenting with different combinations and variations of these herbs can help individuals discover personalized blends that suit their tastes and health goals.

CHAPTER SEVEN

Supporting the Body's Elimination Pathways: Understanding How Juicing Enhances Detox Processes

Detoxification is a natural process by which the body eliminates toxins and waste products to maintain health and vitality. Supporting the body's elimination pathways is essential for effective detoxification, and herbal juicing can play a significant role in enhancing these processes. In this guide, we explore how juicing supports the body's detoxification pathways, including the liver, kidneys, digestive system, skin, and lymphatic system, and promotes overall well-being.

1. Liver Support

The liver is the body's primary detoxification organ, responsible for metabolizing and eliminating toxins from the bloodstream. Herbal juices containing liver-supportive ingredients such as dandelion, milk thistle, turmeric, and beetroot can help enhance liver function, stimulate bile production, and promote the breakdown and elimination of toxins.

2. Kidney Function

The kidneys play a crucial role in filtering waste products and toxins from the blood and excreting them in the form of urine. Hydration is essential for supporting kidney function, and drinking plenty of water and herbal juices helps flush out toxins and promote kidney health. Herbal ingredients such as parsley, cilantro, and lemon can also support kidney function and promote urinary tract health.

3. Digestive Health

A healthy digestive system is vital for effective detoxification, as it facilitates the breakdown and elimination of toxins from the body. Herbal juices containing fiber-rich ingredients such as fruits, vegetables, and herbs support digestive health by promoting regular bowel movements and reducing constipation. Additionally, ingredients like ginger and turmeric can help alleviate digestive discomfort and support gastrointestinal function.

4. Skin Detoxification

The skin is the body's largest organ and plays a crucial role in detoxification through sweat production. Herbal juices containing hydrating ingredients such as cucumber, watermelon, and coconut water can support skin health and promote sweating, aiding in the elimination of toxins through the skin. Additionally, antioxidants found in fruits and vegetables help protect the skin from oxidative damage and promote a healthy complexion.

5. Lymphatic System

The lymphatic system is a network of vessels and lymph nodes that helps remove toxins, waste products, and pathogens from the body. Herbal juices containing lymphatic-supportive ingredients such as ginger, lemon, and cilantro can help stimulate lymphatic circulation, support immune function, and enhance detoxification. Incorporating ingredients like wheatgrass and spirulina can also support lymphatic drainage and promote overall well-being.

6. Alkalizing the Body

Many herbal ingredients used in juicing have alkalizing properties, which help balance the body's pH levels and create an alkaline environment conducive to detoxification. Alkalizing ingredients such as lemon, cucumber, spinach, and kale help neutralize acidity in the body, reduce inflammation, and promote cellular detoxification. By consuming alkalizing herbal juices, individuals can support the body's natural detoxification processes and promote overall health and vitality.

Conclusion

Herbal juicing offers a powerful and effective way to support the body's natural detoxification processes and promote overall well-being. By incorporating liver-supportive ingredients, promoting kidney function, supporting digestive health, aiding skin detoxification, stimulating lymphatic circulation, and alkalizing the body, herbal juices enhance detox processes and promote optimal health. Incorporating a variety of nutrient-rich fruits, vegetables, and herbs into juicing recipes ensures a broad spectrum of vitamins, minerals, antioxidants, and phytochemicals that support detoxification and promote vitality. By embracing herbal juicing as part of a balanced and healthy lifestyle, individuals can support their body's detoxification pathways and enjoy renewed energy, vitality, and well-being.

CHAPTER EIGHT

Detoxification Symptoms and Side Effects: Managing Potential Reactions During the Cleanse

Embarking on a detoxification journey, such as Doctor Barbara's Herbal Juice Detox, can lead to various symptoms and side effects as the body undergoes the process of cleansing and elimination. While these reactions are typically temporary and indicative of the body's healing response, it's essential to understand and manage them effectively to ensure a safe and successful cleanse. In this guide, we explore common detoxification symptoms and side effects and provide strategies for managing them during the cleanse.

1. Headaches

Headaches are a common detoxification symptom that may arise as the body eliminates toxins and adjusts to dietary changes. These headaches can be caused by caffeine withdrawal, dehydration, or the release of stored toxins into the bloodstream. To manage headaches during the cleanse:

- Stay hydrated by drinking plenty of water and herbal teas throughout the day.

- Gradually reduce caffeine intake before starting the cleanse to minimize withdrawal symptoms.

- Practice stress-reduction techniques such as deep breathing, meditation, or gentle exercise to alleviate tension and promote relaxation.

- Apply a cold compress to the forehead or temples to ease headache discomfort.

2. Fatigue

Fatigue is another common side effect of detoxification as the body expends energy to eliminate toxins and support cellular repair. While it's normal to experience some fatigue during the cleanse, severe or prolonged fatigue may indicate the need for adjustments to the detox protocol. To manage fatigue during the cleanse:

- Ensure adequate rest and sleep by prioritizing early bedtime and minimizing exposure to stimulating activities before bed.

- Support energy levels with nutrient-rich herbal juices, whole foods, and hydration throughout the day.

- Incorporate gentle exercise such as walking, yoga, or tai chi to promote circulation, oxygenation, and energy flow in the body.

- Listen to your body and rest when needed, allowing time for the body to recharge and rejuvenate during the cleanse.

3. Digestive Discomfort

Digestive discomfort such as bloating, gas, or constipation may occur as the body adjusts to dietary changes and eliminates toxins. These symptoms may be exacerbated by the increased intake of fiber-rich fruits and vegetables during the cleanse. To manage digestive discomfort during the cleanse:

- Increase fiber intake gradually before starting the cleanse to minimize digestive upset.

- Drink plenty of water and herbal teas to support hydration and promote regular bowel movements.

- Incorporate digestive-friendly herbs such as ginger, peppermint, or fennel into herbal juices to alleviate bloating and gas.

- Eat smaller, more frequent meals to ease digestion and reduce the burden on the digestive system.

4. Skin Breakouts

Skin breakouts or flare-ups may occur during the cleanse as the body eliminates toxins through the skin. These breakouts are often temporary and may indicate that the body is purging impurities and cleansing the skin from within. To manage skin breakouts during the cleanse:

- Maintain a consistent skincare routine using gentle, non-irritating products to cleanse and moisturize the skin.

- Avoid touching or picking at blemishes to prevent further irritation and scarring.

- Support skin health with hydrating herbal juices, antioxidant-rich foods, and adequate hydration throughout the day.

- Consider incorporating skin-supportive herbs such as burdock root, cleavers, or red clover into herbal juices to promote detoxification and skin health.

5. Emotional Changes

Detoxification can also affect emotional well-being, leading to mood swings, irritability, or heightened emotions as the body releases stored toxins and emotions. These emotional changes are a natural part of the cleansing process and may indicate that the body is releasing pent-up stress and tension. To manage emotional changes during the cleanse:

- Practice self-care activities such as meditation, deep breathing, or journaling to promote relaxation and emotional balance.

- Engage in gentle exercise such as yoga or walking to release tension, promote circulation, and support emotional well-being.

- Seek support from friends, family members, or a healthcare professional if experiencing intense emotional reactions during the cleanse.

- Be patient and compassionate with yourself, acknowledging that emotional changes are a normal part of the detoxification process and temporary in nature.

6. Intensity and Duration

It's important to note that detoxification symptoms and side effects can vary in intensity and duration depending on individual factors such as overall health, toxin exposure, and the body's detoxification capacity. While some individuals may experience mild symptoms that resolve quickly, others may experience more intense reactions that persist throughout the cleanse. It's essential to listen to your body, adjust the detox protocol as needed, and seek guidance from a healthcare professional if experiencing severe or prolonged symptoms during the cleanse.

Conclusion

Detoxification symptoms and side effects are a natural part of the cleansing process as the body eliminates toxins and adjusts to dietary changes. By understanding common detoxification reactions and implementing strategies to manage them effectively, individuals can support their body's detoxification journey and promote overall health and well-being during the cleanse. Through hydration, rest, nourishing herbal juices, gentle exercise, and self-care practices, individuals can navigate detoxification symptoms with confidence and experience the transformative benefits of a thorough cleanse.

CHAPTER NINE

Testimonials of Transformation: Inspiring Stories of Individuals Who Have Completed Doctor Barbara's 7-Day Herbal Juice Detox

Embarking on Doctor Barbara's 7-Day Herbal Juice Detox can be a transformative journey towards renewed health, vitality, and well-being. Many individuals have experienced profound changes in their physical, mental, and emotional health after completing the cleanse. In this compilation of testimonials, we share inspiring stories of individuals who have undergone Doctor Barbara's Herbal Juice Detox and emerged with renewed energy, improved digestion, clearer skin, and a greater sense of well-being.

1. Sarah's Journey to Radiant Health

"After years of struggling with fatigue, digestive issues, and skin breakouts, I decided to try Doctor Barbara's Herbal Juice Detox as a last resort. I was skeptical at first, but after completing the cleanse, I was amazed at the results. Not only did I experience a significant increase in energy levels, but my digestion improved, and my skin cleared up dramatically. I feel lighter, more vibrant, and more alive than ever before. Doctor Barbara's Herbal Juice Detox has truly transformed my health and my life."

2. David's Experience of Renewed Vitality

"As someone who leads a busy and stressful lifestyle, I often found myself feeling exhausted, irritable, and rundown. After hearing about Doctor Barbara's Herbal Juice Detox from a friend, I decided to give it a try. I was blown away by the results. Not only did I experience a surge of energy and vitality during the cleanse, but I also noticed improvements in my mood, focus, and overall well-being. Doctor Barbara's Herbal Juice Detox has become an essential part of my self-care routine, and I can't recommend it enough."

3. Emily's Journey to Digestive Wellness

"For years, I struggled with bloating, gas, and digestive discomfort, despite trying countless diets and supplements. I was skeptical that a 7-day herbal juice cleanse could make a difference, but I was willing to give it a try. To my surprise, the results were remarkable. Not only did my digestive symptoms improve significantly during the cleanse, but I also noticed a newfound sense of lightness and clarity. Doctor Barbara's Herbal Juice Detox has helped me reclaim my digestive health and rediscover the joy of eating."

4. Michael's Transformational Journey

"As someone who has struggled with weight management and emotional eating for most of my life, I was desperate for a solution. Doctor Barbara's Herbal Juice Detox offered me a glimmer of hope, and I decided to commit to the cleanse wholeheartedly. The experience was nothing short of transformational. Not only did I shed excess weight and inches from my waistline, but I also gained a newfound sense of self-confidence and empowerment. Doctor Barbara's Herbal Juice Detox has given me the tools and support I need to live a healthier, happier life."

5. Jessica's Journey to Clearer Skin

"As someone who has battled acne for years, I was willing to try anything to clear up my skin. Doctor Barbara's Herbal Juice Detox came highly recommended, so I decided to give it a shot. To my amazement, the results were beyond anything I could have imagined. Not only did my skin clear up significantly during the cleanse, but it also became brighter, smoother, and more radiant. Doctor Barbara's Herbal Juice Detox has given me the confidence to show my skin to the world and embrace my natural beauty."

Conclusion

These testimonials offer a glimpse into the transformative power of Doctor Barbara's 7-Day Herbal Juice Detox. From increased energy and vitality to improved digestion, clearer skin, and a greater sense of well-being, individuals have experienced a wide range of benefits after completing the cleanse. If you're considering embarking on your own detox journey, let these inspiring stories serve as motivation and encouragement to take the first step towards renewed health and vitality with Doctor Barbara's Herbal Juice Detox.

CHAPTER TEN

Post-Detox Maintenance: Strategies for Transitioning Back to Solid Foods and Sustaining Healthful Habits

Completing a detox, such as Doctor Barbara's 7-Day Herbal Juice Detox, marks the end of a transformative journey towards renewed health and vitality. However, transitioning back to solid foods and maintaining healthful habits is crucial for sustaining the benefits of the cleanse in the long term. In this guide, we outline strategies for post-detox maintenance, including gradual reintroduction of solid foods, mindful eating practices, and sustainable lifestyle habits to support ongoing health and well-being.

1. Gradual Reintroduction of Solid Foods

After completing a detox, it's essential to reintroduce solid foods gradually to avoid overwhelming the digestive system and minimize the risk of digestive discomfort or bloating. Start by incorporating easily digestible foods such as steamed vegetables, soups, salads, and lean proteins into your diet. Gradually reintroduce other foods such as whole grains, legumes, nuts, and seeds over the course of several days to allow your body to adjust to solid foods gradually.

2. Mindful Eating Practices

Practicing mindful eating can help you reconnect with your body's hunger and fullness cues, promote healthy eating habits, and prevent overeating or emotional eating. Take time to savor and enjoy each bite, chew food thoroughly, and pay attention to the flavors, textures, and sensations of each meal. Eat slowly, without distractions, and tune in to your body's signals of hunger and satisfaction to guide your eating choices.

3. Balanced Nutrition

Focus on maintaining a balanced and nutrient-rich diet that includes a variety of fruits, vegetables, whole grains, lean proteins, and healthy fats. Aim to fill your plate with colorful fruits and vegetables, incorporate plant-based proteins such as beans, lentils, and tofu, and choose whole grains such as quinoa, brown rice, and oats for sustained energy and satiety. Include sources of healthy fats such as avocado, nuts, seeds, and olive oil to support heart health and brain function.

4. Hydration

Stay hydrated by drinking plenty of water throughout the day to support digestion, detoxification, and overall health. Aim to drink at least 8-10 glasses of water per day, and consider incorporating hydrating beverages such as herbal teas, coconut water, and infused water with fresh fruits and herbs. Limit consumption of sugary beverages, caffeinated drinks, and alcohol, which can dehydrate the body and undermine your health goals.

5. Regular Physical Activity

Maintain an active lifestyle by incorporating regular physical activity into your daily routine. Aim for at least 30 minutes of moderate-intensity exercise most days of the week, such as walking, jogging, cycling, swimming, or yoga. Find activities that you enjoy and make them a priority, whether it's taking a brisk walk outdoors, attending a fitness class, or practicing yoga at home. Regular exercise supports cardiovascular health, strengthens muscles and bones, boosts mood, and enhances overall well-being.

6. Stress Management

Prioritize stress management techniques to support your mental and emotional well-being. Practice relaxation techniques such as deep breathing, meditation, mindfulness, or progressive muscle relaxation to reduce stress levels, promote relaxation, and enhance resilience to stressors. Take time for self-care activities that nourish your mind, body, and spirit, whether it's spending time in nature, practicing hobbies, or connecting with loved ones.

7. Sustainable Lifestyle Habits

Focus on cultivating sustainable lifestyle habits that support your health and well-being in the long term. This includes getting adequate sleep each night, practicing good hygiene, maintaining a healthy weight, and avoiding harmful habits such as smoking or excessive alcohol consumption. Embrace a holistic approach to health that encompasses physical, mental, and emotional well-being, and prioritize self-care practices that promote balance, vitality, and longevity.

By incorporating these strategies for post-detox maintenance into your daily routine, you can sustain the benefits of the cleanse, support ongoing health and well-being, and cultivate a balanced and vibrant lifestyle for the long term. Remember that small, consistent changes over time can lead to significant improvements in your health and quality of life, so be patient, stay committed to your goals, and celebrate your progress along the way.

BONUS: SOME HERBAL REMEDIES TO KNOW

Bio Ferro Tonic:

Definition: Bio Ferro Tonic is a dietary supplement primarily composed of herbs and minerals. It's often marketed as a natural way to support overall health, particularly by promoting blood health and circulation.

Ingredients: Typical ingredients in Bio Ferro Tonic may include a blend of herbs such as burdock root, yellow dock root, sarsaparilla root, and cascara sagrada bark, along with minerals like iron and potassium phosphate.

How to Prepare: Bio Ferro Tonic usually comes in liquid form and is typically taken orally. It's important to follow the instructions on the product label for dosage and administration.

Dosage: The dosage can vary depending on the specific product and individual needs. It's crucial to consult with a healthcare professional or follow the recommended dosage on the product label to avoid potential side effects.

How to Use: Bio Ferro Tonic is often taken by adding the recommended dosage to water or juice and consuming it orally. It's important to shake the bottle well before use and store it according to the manufacturer's instructions.

Side Effects: While Bio Ferro Tonic is generally considered safe when used as directed, some individuals may experience side effects such as digestive discomfort, allergic reactions, or interactions with medications. It's essential to consult with a healthcare provider before starting any new supplement regimen, especially if you have underlying health conditions or are taking medications.

Bladderwrack:

Definition: Bladderwrack is a type of seaweed or marine algae commonly used in traditional medicine and as a dietary supplement. It's known for its potential health benefits, particularly related to thyroid health and weight management.

Ingredients: Bladderwrack contains various nutrients, including iodine, vitamins, minerals, and antioxidants. The primary active components are iodine and fucoidan, a type of carbohydrate found in brown seaweeds.

How to Prepare: Bladderwrack supplements are available in various forms, including capsules, powders, and liquid extracts. They can be taken orally with water or added to smoothies and other beverages.

Dosage: The appropriate dosage of bladderwrack can vary based on factors such as age, health status, and the specific product being used. It's essential to follow the recommended dosage on the product label or consult with a healthcare professional for personalized guidance.

How to Use: Bladderwrack supplements are typically taken orally, either with water or mixed into food or beverages. It's important to follow the instructions on the product label and avoid exceeding the recommended dosage.

Side Effects: While bladderwrack is generally considered safe for most people when used in moderation, excessive intake of iodine from bladderwrack supplements can cause thyroid dysfunction and other adverse effects. Individuals with thyroid disorders, iodine sensitivity, or certain medical conditions should exercise caution and consult with a healthcare provider before using bladderwrack supplements. Common side effects may include digestive upset, allergic reactions, or interactions with medications.

Blood Purifier:

Definition: Blood purifiers are herbal remedies or dietary supplements believed to cleanse or detoxify the blood, often promoting overall health and well-being. They are thought to support the body's natural detoxification processes and improve blood circulation.

Ingredients: Blood purifiers may contain a variety of herbs and botanical extracts known for their purported cleansing and detoxifying properties. Common ingredients include burdock root, red clover, dandelion root, and yellow dock root, among others.

How to Prepare: Blood purifiers are typically available in various forms, including capsules, tablets, powders, and liquid extracts. They are usually taken orally with water or juice, following the recommended dosage on the product label.

Dosage: The dosage of blood purifiers can vary depending on the specific product and individual needs. It's important to adhere to the recommended dosage on the product label or consult with a healthcare professional for personalized guidance.

How to Use: Blood purifiers are typically taken orally, either with water or mixed into beverages. They are often used as part of a detoxification regimen or to support overall health and vitality.

Side Effects: While blood purifiers are generally considered safe for most people when used as directed, some individuals may experience side effects such as digestive discomfort, allergic reactions, or interactions with medications. It's important to consult with a healthcare provider before starting any new supplement regimen, especially if you have underlying health conditions or are taking medications.

Blue Vervain:

Definition: Blue vervain, also known as Verbena hastata, is a perennial herb native to North America. It has been used in traditional medicine for centuries to treat various ailments, including anxiety, insomnia, and digestive issues.

Ingredients: Blue vervain contains several active compounds, including aucubin, verbenalin, and volatile oils. These compounds are believed to contribute to the herb's medicinal properties.

How to Prepare: Blue vervain is typically consumed as a tea or tincture. To make tea, dried blue vervain leaves and flowers are steeped in hot water for several minutes before being strained and consumed. Tinctures are prepared by steeping the herb in alcohol or vinegar to extract its active compounds.

Dosage: The appropriate dosage of blue vervain can vary depending on factors such as age, health status, and the specific preparation being used. It's important to follow the recommended dosage on the product label or consult with a qualified herbalist or healthcare professional for personalized guidance.

How to Use: Blue vervain tea or tincture is typically taken orally. It can be consumed on its own or mixed with honey or other herbal teas for added flavor.

Side Effects: While blue vervain is generally considered safe for most people when used in moderation, excessive intake may cause digestive upset or allergic reactions in some individuals. Pregnant or breastfeeding women should avoid blue vervain due to its potential to stimulate uterine contractions. As with any herbal remedy, it's important to consult with a healthcare provider before using blue vervain, especially if you have underlying health conditions or are taking medications.

Bromide Plus Powder:

Definition: Bromide Plus Powder is a dietary supplement formulated to support thyroid health and promote overall well-being. It typically contains a blend of herbs and minerals that are believed to have beneficial effects on thyroid function.

Ingredients: Bromide Plus Powder often contains a combination of herbs such as bladderwrack, sea moss, and burdock root, along with minerals like iodine and potassium phosphate. These ingredients are thought to support thyroid function and maintain optimal iodine levels in the body.

How to Prepare: Bromide Plus Powder is usually mixed with water or juice to create a drinkable solution. It's important to follow the instructions on the product label for dosage and preparation.

Dosage: The dosage of Bromide Plus Powder can vary depending on the specific product and individual needs. It's crucial to consult with a healthcare professional or follow the recommended dosage on the product label to avoid potential side effects.

How to Use: Bromide Plus Powder is typically taken orally by mixing the recommended dosage with water or juice. It's important to shake or stir the mixture well before consuming it to ensure even distribution of the ingredients.

Side Effects: While Bromide Plus Powder is generally considered safe when used as directed, some individuals may experience side effects such as digestive discomfort or allergic reactions to certain ingredients. It's essential to consult with a healthcare provider before starting any new supplement regimen, especially if you have underlying health conditions or are taking medications.

Bugleweed:

Definition: Bugleweed, also known as Lycopusvirginicus, is a perennial herb native to North America and Europe. It has been used in traditional medicine to treat various conditions, including hyperthyroidism, anxiety, and insomnia.

Ingredients: Bugleweed contains several active compounds, including lithospermic acid, phenolic acids, and flavonoids. These compounds are believed to contribute to the herb's medicinal properties, particularly its ability to regulate thyroid function.

How to Prepare: Bugleweed is commonly consumed as a tea or tincture. To make tea, dried bugleweed leaves and flowers are steeped in hot water for several minutes before being strained and consumed. Tinctures are prepared by steeping the herb in alcohol or vinegar to extract its active compounds.

Dosage: The appropriate dosage of bugleweed can vary depending on factors such as age, health status, and the specific preparation being used. It's important to follow the recommended dosage on the product label or consult with a qualified herbalist or healthcare professional for personalized guidance.

How to Use: Bugleweed tea or tincture is typically taken orally. It can be consumed on its own or mixed with honey or other herbal teas for added flavor.

Side Effects: While bugleweed is generally considered safe for most people when used in moderation, excessive intake may cause digestive upset or allergic reactions in some individuals. Pregnant or breastfeeding women should avoid bugleweed due to its potential to stimulate uterine contractions. As with any herbal remedy, it's important to consult with a healthcare provider before using bugleweed, especially if you have underlying health conditions or are taking medications.

Burdock:

Definition: Burdock, scientifically known as Arctium lappa, is a biennial plant native to Europe and Asia but now found worldwide. It's part of the Asteraceae family and has been used for centuries in traditional medicine and culinary practices.

Ingredients: Burdock contains various nutrients, including carbohydrates, fiber, vitamins (such as vitamin B6, folate, and vitamin C), and minerals (including potassium, magnesium, and manganese). It also contains active compounds such as polyphenols and volatile oils.

How to Prepare: Burdock can be prepared and consumed in various ways. The roots, leaves, and seeds are all utilized for different purposes. The root is commonly used in cooking, herbal teas, tinctures, and supplements, while the leaves and seeds are sometimes used in herbal preparations.

Dosage: The appropriate dosage of burdock root can vary depending on the specific form and intended use. For culinary purposes, there are no strict dosage guidelines, but for supplements or herbal remedies, it's essential to follow the recommended dosage on the product label or consult with a healthcare professional.

How to Use: Burdock root can be used in cooking by peeling, slicing, and adding it to soups, stews, stir-fries, or salads. It can also be brewed into a tea or used to make tinctures or extracts for medicinal purposes. Some people may also take burdock root supplements in capsule or powder form.

Side Effects: While burdock is generally considered safe for most people when consumed in moderate amounts, some individuals may experience allergic reactions or digestive upset. Additionally, burdock may interact with certain medications or have adverse effects in individuals with certain health conditions, such as diabetes or allergies to plants in the Asteraceae family. It's important to consult with a healthcare provider before using burdock, especially if you have underlying health conditions or are taking medications.

Cascara Sagrada:

Definition: Cascara Sagrada, scientifically known as Rhamnus purshiana, is a species of buckthorn native to western North America. It has been used traditionally as a laxative and to promote bowel regularity.

Ingredients: The primary active ingredients in cascara sagrada are anthraquinone glycosides, particularly cascarosides A and B. These compounds stimulate peristalsis in the colon, leading to increased bowel movements.

How to Prepare: Cascara sagrada is typically prepared as an herbal tea, tincture, or capsule. To make tea, dried cascara sagrada bark is steeped in hot water for several minutes before being strained and consumed. Tinctures are prepared by steeping the bark in alcohol to extract its active compounds.

Dosage: The appropriate dosage of cascara sagrada can vary depending on the specific preparation and intended use. It's important to follow the recommended dosage on the product label or consult with a healthcare professional for personalized guidance.

How to Use: Cascara sagrada tea or tincture is typically taken orally. It's important to start with a low dose and gradually increase if needed to avoid potential side effects such as cramping or diarrhea.

Side Effects: Cascara sagrada is considered safe for short-term use when used as directed. However, long-term or excessive use may lead to dependence, electrolyte imbalance, or dehydration. It may also interact with certain medications or have adverse effects in individuals with certain health conditions. It's important to use cascara sagrada under the guidance of a healthcare professional and to discontinue use if any adverse effects occur.

Cell Food:

Definition: Cell Food is a dietary supplement marketed as a highly oxygenating and alkalizing formula. It's claimed to support overall health and vitality by providing essential nutrients and oxygen to the cells.

Ingredients: The exact ingredients of Cell Food can vary depending on the brand, but it typically contains a proprietary blend of minerals, enzymes, electrolytes, and trace elements. Some common ingredients may include purified water, dissolved oxygen, seawater extract, and plant-based enzymes.

How to Prepare: Cell Food is usually available in liquid form and is typically taken orally. It can be consumed directly or diluted in water or juice before consumption.

Dosage: The dosage of Cell Food can vary depending on the specific product and individual needs. It's important to follow the recommended dosage on the product label or consult with a healthcare professional for personalized guidance.

How to Use: Cell Food is typically taken orally, either directly or mixed into water or juice. It's important to shake the bottle well before use and to store it according to the manufacturer's instructions.

Side Effects: Cell Food is generally considered safe for most people when used as directed. However, some individuals may experience mild digestive upset or allergic reactions to certain ingredients. It's essential to consult with a healthcare provider before starting any new supplement regimen, especially if you have underlying health conditions or are taking medications.

Chaparral:

Definition: Chaparral, scientifically known as Larrea tridentata, is a shrub native to the southwestern United States and northern

Mexico. It has been used for centuries by Native American tribes for its medicinal properties and is commonly used in herbal medicine today.

Ingredients: Chaparral contains several bioactive compounds, including nordihydroguaiaretic acid (NDGA), flavonoids, lignans, and volatile oils. NDGA is believed to be the primary active compound responsible for many of chaparral's therapeutic effects.

How to Prepare: Chaparral can be prepared and consumed in various forms, including teas, tinctures, capsules, and topical preparations. To make tea, dried chaparral leaves are steeped in hot water for several minutes before being strained and consumed. Tinctures are prepared by steeping the herb in alcohol or vinegar to extract its active compounds.

Dosage: The appropriate dosage of chaparral can vary depending on the specific form and intended use. It's important to follow the recommended dosage on the product label or consult with a healthcare professional for personalized guidance.

How to Use: Chaparral tea or tincture is typically taken orally. It can also be applied topically to the skin for certain conditions. It's important to use chaparral products as directed and to discontinue use if any adverse effects occur.

Side Effects: Chaparral is generally considered safe for most people when used in moderate amounts. However, excessive intake or prolonged use may lead to liver toxicity or other adverse effects. It may also interact with certain medications or have adverse effects in individuals with certain health conditions. It's important to use chaparral under the guidance of a healthcare professional and to discontinue use if any adverse effects occur.

Cocolmeca:

Definition: Cocolmeca, also known as Smilax ornata or sarsaparilla, is a flowering vine native to Mexico and Central America. It has been used traditionally in Mexican and Central American folk medicine for its purported medicinal properties.

Ingredients: Cocolmeca contains various bioactive compounds, including saponins, flavonoids, and plant sterols. These compounds are believed to contribute to the herb's medicinal properties, including its potential as a diuretic, blood purifier, and anti-inflammatory agent.

How to Prepare: Cocolmeca is commonly prepared and consumed as an herbal tea or decoction. To make tea, dried cocolmeca roots or leaves are steeped in hot water for several minutes before being strained and consumed. Decoctions involve boiling the roots or leaves in water to extract their active compounds.

Dosage: The appropriate dosage of cocolmeca can vary depending on factors such as age, health status, and the specific preparation being used. It's important to follow the recommended dosage on the product label or consult with a qualified herbalist or healthcare professional for personalized guidance.

How to Use: Cocolmeca tea or decoction is typically taken orally. It can also be used topically for certain skin conditions. It's important to use cocolmeca products as directed and to discontinue use if any adverse effects occur.

Side Effects: Cocolmeca is generally considered safe for most people when used in moderate amounts. However, excessive intake may lead to digestive upset or other adverse effects. It may also interact with certain medications or have adverse effects in individuals with certain health conditions. It's important to use cocolmeca under the guidance of a healthcare professional and to discontinue use if any adverse effects occur.

Contribo:

Definition: Contribo, also known as Aristolochiatrilobata, is a vine native to the Caribbean and Central America. It has been used traditionally in folk medicine for various purposes, including as a remedy for digestive issues, inflammation, and pain relief.

Ingredients: Contribo contains several bioactive compounds, including aristolochic acids, flavonoids, and alkaloids. These compounds are believed to contribute to the herb's medicinal properties, including its potential as an anti-inflammatory and analgesic agent.

How to Prepare: Contribo is typically prepared and consumed as an herbal tea or decoction. To make tea, dried contribo leaves or stems are steeped in hot water for several minutes before being strained and consumed. Decoctions involve boiling the leaves or stems in water to extract their active compounds.

Dosage: The appropriate dosage of contribo can vary depending on factors such as age, health status, and the specific preparation being used. It's important to follow the recommended dosage on the product label or consult with a qualified herbalist or healthcare professional for personalized guidance.

How to Use: Contribo tea or decoction is typically taken orally. It's important to use contribo products as directed and to discontinue use if any adverse effects occur.

Side Effects: Contribo contains aristolochic acids, which have been associated with serious adverse effects, including kidney damage and cancer. Due to these safety concerns, the use of contribo is highly discouraged, and it's important to avoid products containing aristolochic acids. Individuals should seek alternative remedies for their health needs.

Dandelion Root:

Definition: Dandelion, scientifically known as Taraxacum officinale, is a common flowering plant found worldwide. While often considered a pesky weed, dandelion has a long history of use in traditional medicine for its various health benefits.

Ingredients: Dandelion root contains several bioactive compounds, including sesquiterpene lactones, triterpenes, flavonoids, and polysaccharides. These compounds are believed to contribute to the herb's medicinal properties, including its potential as a diuretic, digestive aid, and liver tonic.

How to Prepare: Dandelion root can be prepared and consumed in various forms, including teas, tinctures, capsules, and extracts. To make tea, dried dandelion root is steeped in hot water for several minutes before being strained and consumed. Tinctures are prepared by steeping the root in alcohol or vinegar to extract its active compounds.

Dosage: The appropriate dosage of dandelion root can vary depending on factors such as age, health status, and the specific preparation being used. It's important to follow the recommended dosage on the product label or consult with a qualified herbalist or healthcare professional for personalized guidance.

How to Use: Dandelion root tea, tincture, or capsules are typically taken orally. It's important to use dandelion root products as directed and to discontinue use if any adverse effects occur.

Side Effects: Dandelion root is generally considered safe for most people when used in moderate amounts. However, some individuals may experience allergic reactions or digestive upset. It may also interact with certain medications or have adverse effects in individuals with certain health conditions. It's important to use dandelion root under the guidance of a healthcare professional and to discontinue use if any adverse effects occur.

Green Food Plus:

Definition: Green Food Plus is a dietary supplement formulated to provide a concentrated source of nutrients derived from various green plants. It's designed to support overall health and well-being by delivering essential vitamins, minerals, antioxidants, and phytonutrients.

Ingredients: Green Food Plus typically contains a blend of powdered green vegetables, grasses, algae, and other plant-based ingredients. Common ingredients may include wheatgrass, barley grass, spirulina, chlorella, alfalfa, kale, spinach, and broccoli, among others.

How to Prepare: Green Food Plus is usually available in powder form and can be mixed with water, juice, or smoothies. It's important to follow the recommended dosage on the product label and to consume it as part of a balanced diet.

Dosage: The appropriate dosage of Green Food Plus can vary depending on the specific product and individual needs. It's important to follow the recommended dosage on the product label or consult with a healthcare professional for personalized guidance.

How to Use: Green Food Plus powder is typically mixed with water, juice, or smoothies and consumed orally. It's often taken once or twice daily, preferably with meals, to maximize nutrient absorption.

Side Effects: Green Food Plus is generally considered safe for most people when used as directed. However, some individuals may experience digestive upset or allergic reactions to certain ingredients. It's important to consult with a healthcare provider before starting any new supplement regimen, especially if you have underlying health conditions or are taking medications.

Guaco:

Definition: Guaco, also known as Mikania cordata or Mikania glomerata, is a medicinal plant native to Central and South America. It has a long history of use in traditional medicine for its potential therapeutic properties.

Ingredients: Guaco contains several bioactive compounds, including coumarins, flavonoids, tannins, and saponins. These compounds are believed to contribute to the herb's medicinal properties, including its potential as an expectorant, anti-inflammatory, and antispasmodic agent.

How to Prepare: Guaco is typically prepared and consumed as an herbal tea or infusion. To make tea, dried guaco leaves are steeped in hot water for several minutes before being strained and consumed.

Dosage: The appropriate dosage of guaco can vary depending on factors such as age, health status, and the specific preparation being used. It's important to follow the recommended dosage on the product label or consult with a qualified herbalist or healthcare professional for personalized guidance.

How to Use: Guaco tea is typically taken orally. It can be consumed on its own or mixed with honey or other herbal teas for added flavor.

Side Effects: Guaco is generally considered safe for most people when used in moderate amounts. However, some individuals may experience allergic reactions or digestive upset. It may also interact with certain medications or have adverse effects in individuals with certain health conditions. It's important to use guaco under the guidance of a healthcare professional and to discontinue use if any adverse effects occur.

Herban Iron:

Definition: Herban Iron is a dietary supplement designed to provide an easily absorbable form of iron to support healthy iron levels in the body. It's particularly beneficial for individuals with iron deficiency or anemia.

Ingredients: Herban Iron typically contains iron in the form of ferrous bisglycinate, which is a highly bioavailable and gentle form of iron that is less likely to cause digestive upset or constipation compared to other forms of iron. It may also contain other ingredients such as vitamin C to enhance iron absorption.

How to Prepare: Herban Iron is usually available in capsule or liquid form. Capsules are taken orally with water, while liquid forms may be mixed with water or juice before consumption. It's important to follow the recommended dosage on the product label.

Dosage: The appropriate dosage of Herban Iron depends on factors such as age, gender, and the severity of iron deficiency. It's important to consult with a healthcare professional to determine the correct dosage for individual needs.

How to Use: Herban Iron capsules are typically taken orally with water, while liquid forms may be mixed with water or juice before consumption. It's important to take Herban Iron as directed and to avoid taking it with dairy products, antacids, or other substances that may interfere with iron absorption.

Side Effects: While Herban Iron is generally considered safe for most people when used as directed, some individuals may experience mild side effects such as gastrointestinal discomfort or constipation. It's important to consult with a healthcare professional before starting any new supplement regimen, especially if you have underlying health conditions or are taking medications.

Hydrangea:

Definition: Hydrangea, scientifically known as Hydrangea arborescens, is a flowering shrub native to North America. It has been used traditionally in herbal medicine for its potential diuretic and anti-inflammatory properties.

Ingredients: Hydrangea contains several bioactive compounds, including saponins, flavonoids, and glycosides. These compounds are believed to contribute to the herb's medicinal properties, including its potential as a diuretic, kidney tonic, and anti-inflammatory agent.

How to Prepare: Hydrangea root is typically prepared and consumed as an herbal tea or tincture. To make tea, dried hydrangea root is steeped in hot water for several minutes before being strained and consumed. Tinctures are prepared by steeping the root in alcohol or vinegar to extract its active compounds.

Dosage: The appropriate dosage of hydrangea can vary depending on factors such as age, health status, and the specific preparation being used. It's important to follow the recommended dosage on the product label or consult with a qualified herbalist or healthcare professional for personalized guidance.

How to Use: Hydrangea tea or tincture is typically taken orally. It's important to use hydrangea products as directed and to discontinue use if any adverse effects occur.

Side Effects: Hydrangea is generally considered safe for most people when used in moderate amounts. However, some individuals may experience digestive upset or allergic reactions. It may also interact with certain medications or have adverse effects in individuals with certain health conditions. It's important to use hydrangea under the guidance of a healthcare professional and to discontinue use if any adverse effects occur.

Irish Moss:

Definition: Irish Moss, scientifically known as Chondrus crispus, is a species of red algae or seaweed native to the Atlantic coastlines of Europe and North America. It has been used for centuries in traditional Irish and Scottish cuisine, as well as in herbal medicine.

Ingredients: Irish Moss is rich in various nutrients, including iodine, sulfur compounds, vitamins (such as vitamin A, vitamin K, and vitamin B12), minerals (including calcium, magnesium, potassium, and sodium), and polysaccharides (such as carrageenan). These nutrients are believed to contribute to the herb's potential health benefits.

How to Prepare: Irish Moss is typically prepared by soaking it in water to rehydrate and soften it before use. It can be added to soups, stews, smoothies, desserts, and other dishes as a thickening agent or nutritional supplement.

Dosage: The appropriate dosage of Irish Moss can vary depending on factors such as age, health status, and the specific preparation being used. It's important to follow recipes or guidelines for culinary use and to consult with a healthcare professional for guidance on using Irish Moss as a dietary supplement.

How to Use: Irish Moss can be used in culinary applications to add thickness and nutritional value to dishes. It can also be consumed as a dietary supplement in the form of capsules, powders, or extracts.

Side Effects: Irish Moss is generally considered safe for most people when consumed in moderate amounts as part of a balanced diet. However, some individuals may be allergic to seaweed or carrageenan, a compound found in Irish Moss that is used as a food additive. It's important to discontinue use if any adverse effects occur and to consult with a healthcare professional if you have any concerns.

Irish Sea Moss:

Definition: Irish Sea Moss is a term often used interchangeably with Irish Moss, referring to the same species of red algae, Chondrus crispus. It's harvested from the rocky shores of the Atlantic coastlines of Europe and North America.

Ingredients: Irish Sea Moss shares the same nutritional profile as Irish Moss, containing iodine, vitamins, minerals, and polysaccharides. It's valued for its potential health benefits, including supporting thyroid function, boosting immune health, and promoting digestion.

How to Prepare: Irish Sea Moss is prepared in the same way as Irish Moss, by soaking it in water to rehydrate and soften it before use. It can be used in culinary applications or consumed as a dietary supplement.

Dosage: The dosage of Irish Sea Moss depends on the form and intended use. As a dietary supplement, it's important to follow the recommended dosage on the product label or consult with a healthcare professional for personalized guidance.

How to Use: Irish Sea Moss can be used in various culinary applications, including soups, smoothies, desserts, and sauces. It can also be consumed as a dietary supplement in the form of capsules, powders, or extracts.

Side Effects: Similar to Irish Moss, Irish Sea Moss is generally considered safe for most people when consumed in moderate amounts. However, individuals with seaweed allergies or sensitivities to carrageenan should exercise caution. It's important to discontinue use if any adverse effects occur and to consult with a healthcare professional if you have any concerns.

Lymphalin:

Definition: Lymphalin is a herbal supplement formulated to support lymphatic system health. The lymphatic system plays a crucial role in immune function and waste removal in the body, and Lymphalin is designed to promote its proper function.

Ingredients: Lymphalin typically contains a blend of herbs and botanical extracts known for their traditional use in supporting lymphatic system health. Common ingredients may include cleavers, red clover, echinacea, burdock root, and calendula, among others.

How to Prepare: Lymphalin is usually available in capsule or liquid form. Capsules are taken orally with water, while liquid forms may be mixed with water or juice before consumption. It's important to follow the recommended dosage on the product label.

Dosage: The appropriate dosage of Lymphalin can vary depending on the specific product and individual needs. It's important to follow the recommended dosage on the product label or consult with a healthcare professional for personalized guidance.

How to Use: Lymphalin capsules are typically taken orally with water, while liquid forms may be mixed with water or juice before consumption. It's often recommended to take Lymphalin on an empty stomach for optimal absorption.

Side Effects: Lymphalin is generally considered safe for most people when used as directed. However, some individuals may experience mild side effects such as gastrointestinal discomfort or allergic reactions to certain ingredients. It's important to consult with a healthcare provider before starting any new supplement regimen, especially if you have underlying health conditions or are taking medications.

Manjakani:

Definition: Manjakani, also known as Quercus infectoria or oak gall, is a natural substance derived from the oak tree. It has been used for centuries in traditional medicine for its potential health benefits, particularly for women's health and vaginal tightening.

Ingredients: Manjakani contains various bioactive compounds, including tannins, flavonoids, and gallic acid. These compounds are believed to contribute to the herb's medicinal properties, including its potential as an astringent and antiseptic agent.

How to Prepare: Manjakani is typically available in powder, capsule, or liquid extract form. It can be taken orally or used topically depending on the intended use. For vaginal tightening, manjakani may be applied topically as a gel or inserted into the vagina in capsule form.

Dosage: The appropriate dosage of manjakani can vary depending on factors such as age, health status, and the specific preparation being used. It's important to follow the recommended dosage on the product label or consult with a qualified herbalist or healthcare professional for personalized guidance.

How to Use: Manjakani can be taken orally or used topically depending on the intended use. It's important to use manjakani products as directed and to discontinue use if any adverse effects occur.

Side Effects: Manjakani is generally considered safe for most people when used in moderate amounts. However, some individuals may experience allergic reactions or skin irritation when used topically. It's important to use manjakani under the guidance of a healthcare professional and to discontinue use if any adverse effects occur.

THE END

www.ingramcontent.com/pod-product-compliance
Lightning Source LLC
Chambersburg PA
CBHW081845250726
48659CB00008B/2614